Rapid Weight Loss Hypnosis Crash Course

A Complete Compilation Of All The Tips To Weight Loss With Self-Hypnosis And Meditation To Stop Emotional Eating

Self Help for Women Academy

Rapid Weight Loss Hypnosis Crash Course

© Copyright 2021 by Self Help for Women Academy - All rights reserved.

The following Book is reproduced below with the goal of providing information that is as accurate and reliable as possible. Regardless, purchasing this Book can be seen as consent to the fact that both the publisher and the author of this book are in no way experts on the topics discussed within and that any recommendations or suggestions that are made herein are for entertainment purposes only. Professionals should be consulted as needed prior to undertaking any of the action endorsed herein.

This declaration is deemed fair and valid by both the American Bar Association and the Committee of Publishers Association and is legally binding throughout the United States.

Furthermore, the transmission, duplication, or reproduction of any of the following work including specific information will be considered an illegal act irrespective of if it is done electronically or in print. This extends to creating a secondary or tertiary copy of the work or a recorded copy and is only allowed with the express written consent from the Publisher. All additional right reserved.

The information in the following pages is broadly considered a truthful and accurate account of facts and as such, any inattention, use, or misuse of the information in question by the reader will render any resulting actions solely under their purview. There are no scenarios in which the publisher or the original author of this work can be in any fashion deemed liable for any hardship or damages that may befall them after undertaking information described herein.

Additionally, the information in the following pages is intended only for informational purposes and should thus be thought of as universal. As befitting its nature, it is presented without assurance regarding its prolonged validity or interim quality. Trademarks that are mentioned are done without written consent and can in no way be considered an endorsement from the trademark holder.

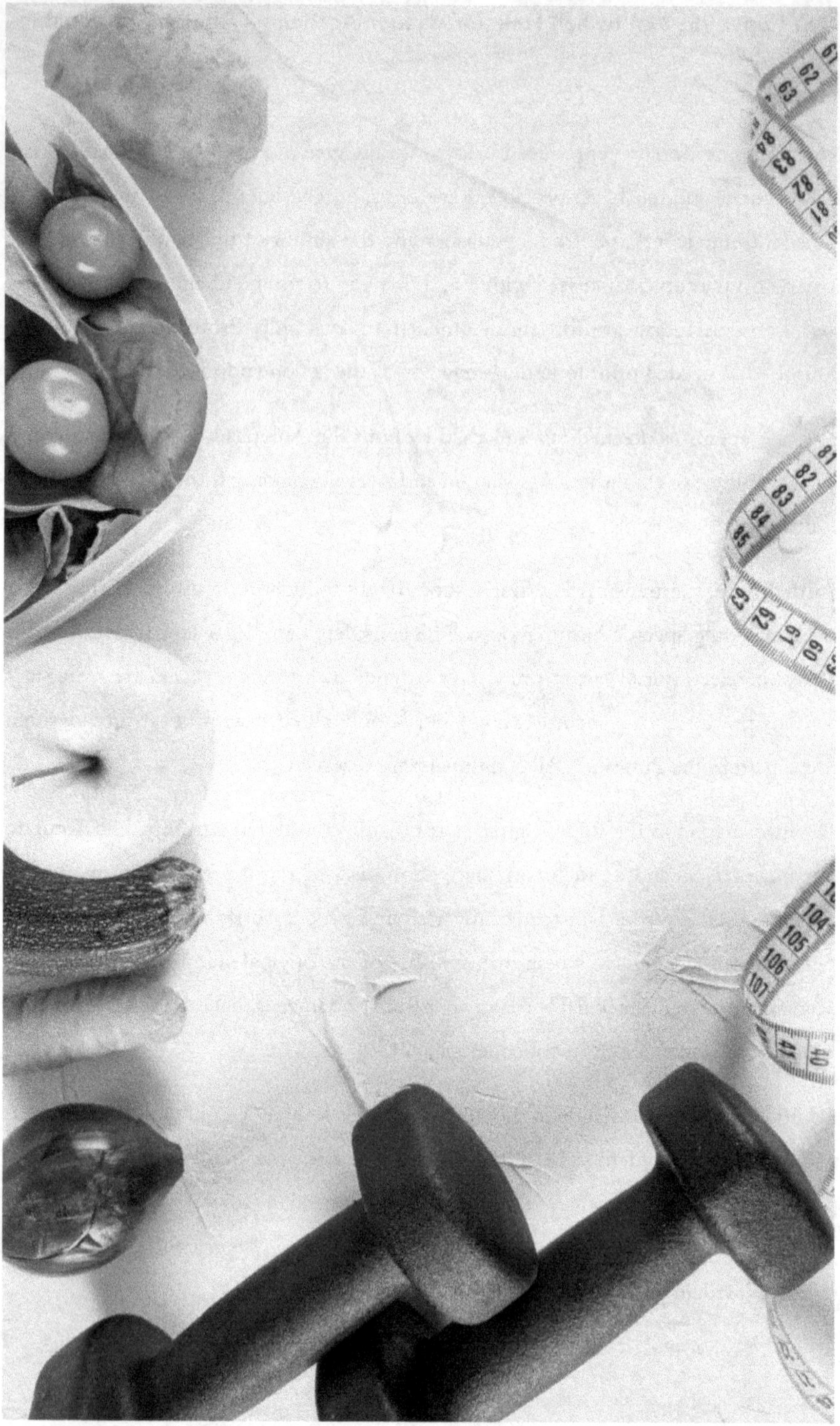

Table of Contents

INTRODUCTION 8
   BASICS TO LEARN TO MEDITATE 9

CHAPTER 1. EAT HEALTHY WITH SUBLIMINAL HYPNOSIS 12
   SUBLIMINAL 12
   SCIENTIFIC RESEARCH ON SUBLIMINAL MESSAGES 17
   THEY HELP QUIT SMOKING 18
   THE MIND CAN HEAR SUBLIMINAL AUDIO MESSAGES 18

CHAPTER 2. LOSING WEIGHT AND EATING HEALTHILY 20
   IMPROVE STUDY SKILLS 21
   SUBLIMINAL MESSAGES TO IMPROVE LEARNING ABILITY 22
   THEY CURE AGORAPHOBIA 23
   PRECISION IN DARTS PLAY 24
   STRONG REACTIONS TO SUBCONSCIOUS MESSAGES 24
   SUBLIMINAL MESSAGES REDUCE SHOPLIFTING 25
   THE POWER OF SUBLIMINAL STIMULUS 26

CHAPTER 3. IDENTIFY NEW WAYS TO COPE WITH STRESS 28
   THE CAUSES OF STRESS 28
   ACUTE STRESS GIVES US "SUPERPOWERS" 29
   CHRONIC STRESS HARMS THE QUALITY OF OUR LIVES 30
   EUSTRESS AND DISTRESS 30
      Stress Is Not Necessarily Negative 30
   HOW TO MANAGE STRESS IN 6 STRATEGIES 31
      Give Priority to What Is Important and Not to What Is Urgent 32
   STRESS CAN BE MANAGED 32
      Knowing Stress 33
   PHYSICAL STRESSORS 34
      Environmental 34
      Physiological 34
   MENTAL STRESSORS 35
      Cognitive 35
      Emotional and Social 35
      Recognize 36
      Manage 36
   YOUR COPING STYLE 37

Some Actions That Work to Prevent and Manage Stress...............38
How to Fight Stress...............39
Awareness...............40
Dealing With Stress...............41
Exercise...............41
Diaphragm Respiration...............42
Meditation...............43
Relaxation Techniques...............43
Sleep Hygiene...............44
Maintaining Social Relationships...............45
How to Manage Stress Through the Act...............45
How to Manage Stress...............46
How to Manage Stress According to the ACT...............47
Managing Stress Through Mindfulness...............48
Fighting Stress Causes Symptoms and Remedies...............49
Sources of Stress...............49
Eliminate Daily Stress on 10 Tips...............53
Foods to Combat Stress...............53
Reduce Stress With a Hot Bath...............55
How to Decrease Stress With a Pet...............55
How to Overcome Stress by Spending Time Outdoors...............56
How to Drain Stress With Art...............57
How to Combat Psychological Stress...............57
How to Reduce Stress With Music...............57
How to Get Rid of Stress With Writing...............58
Reduce Stress With Sexual Activity...............58
How to Manage Stress With Humor...............58
How to Relieve Stress With Prosociality...............59
Fighting Stress With Sport...............59
How a Professional Can Help You Fight Stress...............60
Relaxation Techniques...............60

CHAPTER 4. GET BACK ON TRACK...............62

Don't Bite Any More Than You Can Chew...............63
Concrete Extract...............63
Become a Self-Care Expert...............64
6 Ways to Stabilize Weight Loss...............64
Avoid Carb Creep...............65
Eat According to Your Hunger...............66
Exercise...............67
Try Ketosis...............68

CHAPTER 5. FIRST OF ALL, WHAT IS HYPNOSIS?...............70

Hypnosis for Weight Loss: Applications and Benefits...............71

The Benefits of Hypnosis for Weight Loss *72*
Hypnosis Increases the Ability to Change *72*
But Does Hypnosis Work For Weight Loss? *73*
Who Should Use Hypnosis for Weight Loss? *74*
How Can I Apply Hypnosis for Weight Loss? *74*

CHAPTER 6. LOSING WEIGHT WITH HYPNOSIS: THE TRUTH ABOUT THIS PRACTICE SPREAD ABROAD 76

Hypnosis as Relaxation 76
How to Lose Weight through Hypnosis—We Aim For the Goal 77
Set the Goal 77
Let's Focus on the Goal 78
Let's Define the Points 78

CHAPTER 7. PHYSICAL HUNGER AND EMOTIONAL HUNGER 80

3 Ways to Differentiate Physical Hunger from Emotional 82
Where It Manifests *83*
The Type of Food *83*
Time *84*
How to Differentiate and Manage Your Emotional Hunger 84
What Happens to Your Body When You Are Hungry? 86

CONCLUSION 87

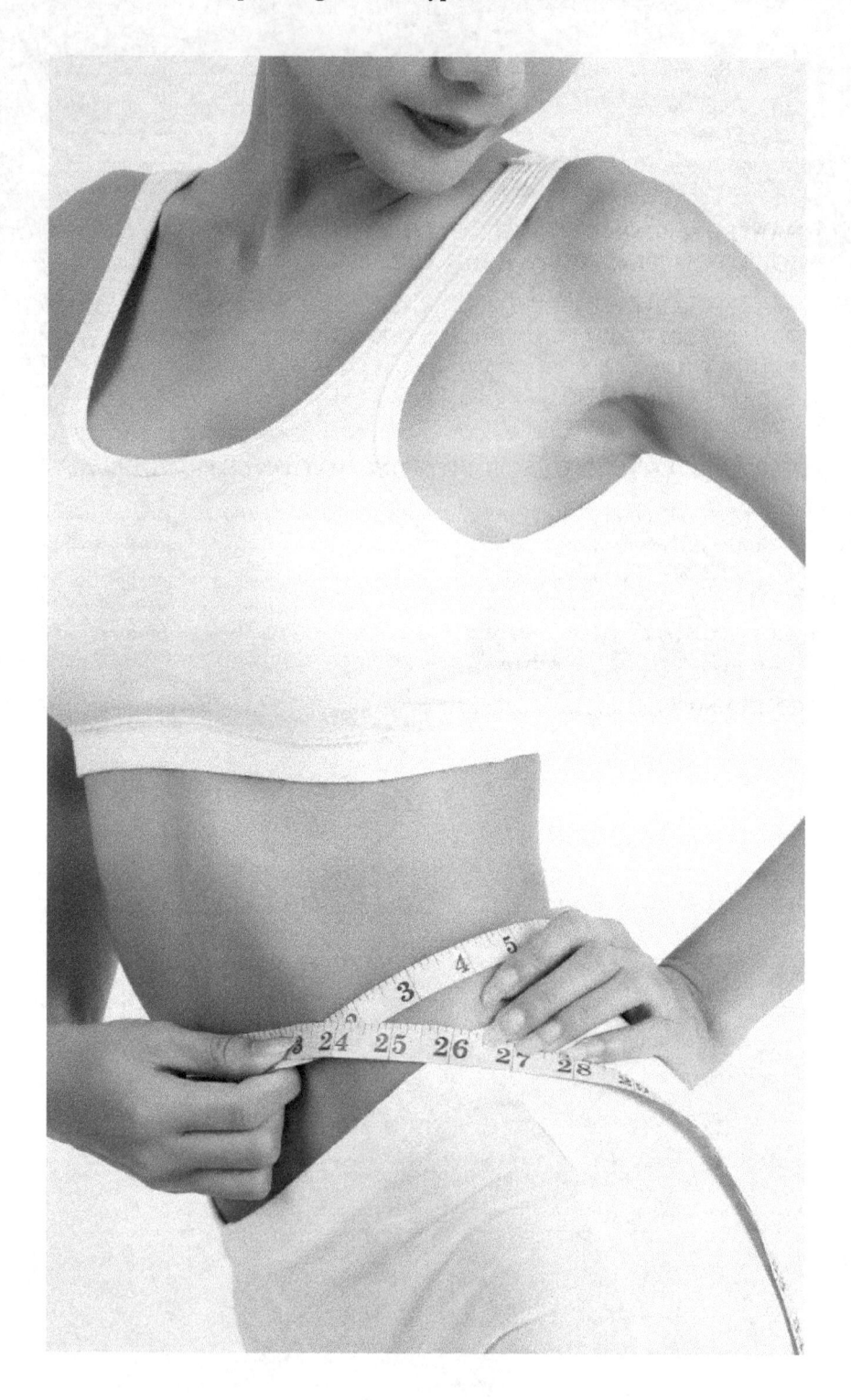

Introduction

What would you answer if we told you that just by closing your eyes and breathing, you could lose weight? What if we revealed that you don't have to eat lettuce and spend hours on gym machines to get to a healthy weight? Directed meditation can help us fight insomnia and reduce stress, but it can also control our appetite, especially when we feel insatiable. The key is to eat consciously. Here are some solutions that can help you achieve it.

1. Before eating, take a second to look at your plate, then examine your food, and think about where it came from and how it got to your table.

2. Pick up the fork, scoop up some food, then put it in front of your face before eating. You will feel the saliva begin to accumulate, and you will feel more conscious about what you will eat.

3. When you are aware of what you are about to consume, eat a little, focus on your tongue, how it works while you eat.

4. Swallow your food, put down your fork, and take a deep breath. These four steps will help you eat mindfully, meditatively, and focus on what you are consuming.

How to tolerate the urge to eat something that we should not eat? Meditation also helps us tolerate pain, visualize it, and let it go. Therefore, if you are trying to lose weight and you are faced with your favorite temptation, for example, a chocolate bar, take the following steps:

1. Look at the chocolate bar

2. Recognize it as a temptation, as something you would like to eat but would be an obstacle to your goals.

3. Visualize it as a wish and let it go away from you.

If you are going through a day full of anxieties, and you feel that at any minute, you will start eating without thinking, then practice meditative breathing, inhaling in four beats, holding in four beats, and exhaling in four beats.

Basics to Learn to Meditate

This week we spoke with Patricio Lagos, yoga instructor, and director of the trends blog Ansia.cl. He gave us some recommendations to learn to meditate and to use meditation to control anxiety and appetite.

But: What does it take to meditate? Can anyone do it?

PL: All you need is the intention to want to do it, to give yourself the time and space for it. It is not a race or competition. It has to be done willingly, relax, and enjoy.

Yes, anyone can do it, and if you have trouble sitting on the floor for a while, don't worry, you can do it sitting in a chair. The main thing is to be comfortable and relaxed. Although you can meditate lying down, remember that the idea is not to sleep, but be present and attentive.

In your experience, what are the benefits of meditation, and how could it help you maintain a proper weight and avoid overeating?

PL: Meditation is a practice that helps you gain talent to guide the flow of your thoughts. If we talk about taking care of your weight and avoiding overeating, the state of relaxation that meditation produces will lower your anxiety level, leading to bad eating habits. After meditation, the mind is in a state of greater clarity, a state from which we are guided towards naturally beneficial behaviors for our body. When the mind is silenced, the wise voice of the body makes itself heard.

But: If we are trying to eat healthily and face a bar of chocolate or other temptation, how could meditation help us stay in line?

When meditation is done a constant practice, the clarity you get is also based on your decisions and habits of thought and behavior. Don't make chocolate or other temptation your enemy. You have to make peace with how things are because when you stop fighting, it is easier to move in the direction you want to go. Be patient with yourself. You are where you are supposed to be, and you are doing very well.

Give it a try, and you will see how meditation will help you control your weight!

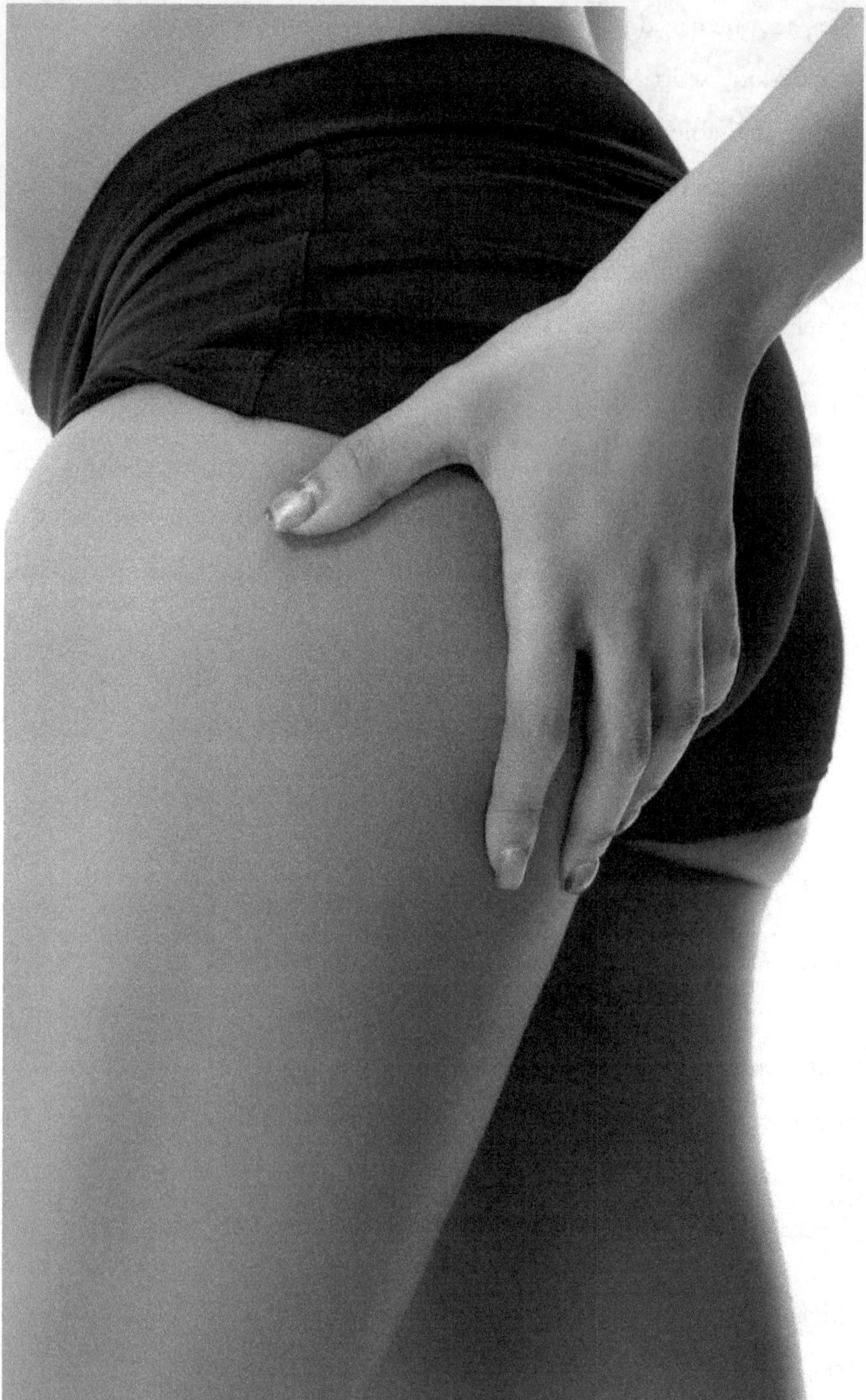

Chapter 1.
Eat Healthy With Subliminal Hypnosis

Subliminal

In the film Matrix, the subliminal message stands out with the increased publicity in the background. The subliminal message is information that is presented in such a way that it is not perceived at a conscious level.

The stimulus sent would directly reach the unconscious part of our brain without the person being able to become aware of it.

They can be sounds, words, phrases, with intensity below the conscious perceptual threshold or interspersed between music and other sounds.

These can be hidden images within other images or representations, such as short sequences between frames in a film.

Therefore, exposure to subliminal information can be so short as to circumvent the possibility of conscious processing, but even if not perceived as such subliminal images or messages can evoke emotional and behavioral responses.

Subliminal derives from the Latin sub limen, i.e., below the threshold level. When used deliberately, it is part of persuasion strategies, which have advertising as a social paradigm.

I considered it useful to integrate this site's information by mentioning the subliminal, which shares hypnosis at the unconscious level of operation.

Although it can be used as a treatment tool, subliminal isolation without the sphere's rational involvement has a temporary clinical efficacy. Its use in other spheres and illegal, violating free will, often produces effects not required by the subject and above all undesirable but not always clearly identifiable.

Marshall Mc Luhan's theories provide a rational basis for the influence of subliminal messages. According to the author, the perception of the reality surrounding us occurs in its entirety with instantaneous press och storage. However, only a small part of the stimuli reaches a level of awareness, and in longer times, most remain fixed in some way in unconscious memory. Our minds' unconscious part is identified with the oldest nerve structures in our brains, which can decisively orient and influence our conscious behavior.

Therefore, it is possible to select stimuli capable of circumventing the rational sphere and staring into unconscious memory with appropriate techniques. Conscious and unconscious perception is shown to act simultaneously but with completely independent dynamics that can lead to opposite effects.

Advertising uses many persuasive tools simultaneously. It must attract attention, stimulate curiosity, and facilitate learning using those stimuli that are closest to the consumer's needs, but not only.

Advertising also induces new values and desires that best accord with its function: INCREASE SALES!

For this reason, it repeatedly flaunts unbridled luxury, abundance, power, money, prestige, success, beauty, sexuality, creating new stereotypes related to ways of life, with a distorted vision of everyday reality, in which purely external, "aesthetic" elements dominate in a context of linear carefreeness.

Subliminal messages proper have also been used to enhance the persuasive effect in advertising. One of the most famous examples was coca-cola, which indirectly, through increased sales, demonstrated this type of message's strength.

In Italy, Law 223 of 1990 expressly prohibits the transmission of subliminal messages, but their use is demonstrated in numerous circumstances and questionable purposes.

The following part was taken from the www.ccsg.com. I refer to this for further insights and curiosities, particularly for the auditory subliminal messages; its website is a vast and orderly collection.

One of the first attempts to influence the unconscious took place in 1956 and was carried out by an unknown advertising agent named James Vicary, owner of the subliminal projection company.

After regularly applying for the patent, James Vicary, head of the subliminal projection company, sought customers interested in using equipment that would project a message of the "hungry" type to a film screen every five seconds for only $1/3000°$ of a second. Eat popcorn! (Are you hungry? Eat popcorn!); or drink coke! (Drink coca-cola!)

In Fort Lee, New Jersey, a movie theater used this equipment for six weeks while the movie Picnic was being screened, and sales increased swirling: popcorn by 37.5% and Coca-Cola by 38%. Still, the cinema declined to provide further details about the experiment. The following year, the Precon Process and Equipment Corporation was formed. Its stated "manufacturing sector" consisted of inserting subliminal messages in films, bars, and advertising signs. The company's staff included a psychologist and a neurologist with a degree in engineering. They claimed to have doubled, by exclusively subliminal methods, the consumption of an advertised drink.

The results of Dr. Hal Becker, a Louisiana electronic medicine researcher from prestigious universities such as Tulane, Princeton, and George Washington University, and author of at least forty articles on subliminal appeared in scientific journals, were compelling.

Becker, after having held important positions for 27 years as a specialist in biomedical communication and behavioral engineering, within the University Medical School of Tulane, he managed, thanks also to the allocation of funds for his research, equal to one million dollars, in the development of sophisticated equipment called "tachistoscope," a machine capable of flashing images at an interval of 3-10 seconds without the viewer seeing it.

Through it, this scientist, an expert in subliminal communications, initially wanted to project in the course of flash television broadcasts containing the phrase: "drive safely"! ("guide with caution"). In 1978, the aforementioned electronic medicine researcher, Dr. Becker, developed a mysterious device that he called Bec mark iv digital audio subliminal processor or simply a little black box.

It was an updated version of the tachistoscope consisting of a tape player capable of receiving, mixing, and transmitting an audio signal from two separate sources, one of which was perceptible only at a subliminal level.

Dr. Becker's invention found use in the anti-theft industry conducted in at least 37 U.S. supermarkets. Time magazine reported that hidden in the ubiquitous background music, and messages were inserted with phrases repeated 9,000 times an hour, at a very low volume of the genre: "Be honest, do not steal, I am honest, I will not steal. Don't steal. I'm honest; I will not steal.' Also, it is believed that this device has been and still is being used by many shops, also for persuasive purposes.

Asked about the serious violations of freedom of choice resulting from the application of his findings, Becker defended himself by stating: "I don't see why there should be no thought conditioners when air conditioners exist."

Scientific Research on Subliminal Messages

We are often asked more evidence about subliminal messages, and we are asked a lot of skeptical questions from people who have already experienced these kinds of messages about themselves.

So here's a page where we've put in a lot of studies that have been done on subliminal messages over the last 30 years:

Ariam, S. and Siller, J. "Effects of Subliminal Oneness Stimuli in Hebrew on Academic Performance of Israeli High School Student" Journal of Abnormal Psychology (1982):

- Tenth-year students were texted in Jews saying, "Mom and I are one," "My teacher and I are one," and "People walk down the street" (a neutral statement). These students have received these messages four times a week for six weeks.

- Six weeks later, students who had been exposed to the subliminal statement "Mom and I are one" scored higher in the math exam than other groups of students.

Psychologists argue that messages like "mom and I are one" increase students' self-confidence and help them learn. Interestingly, when the messages were revealed, and the students were aware of what they were receiving, the messages' effect vanished, demonstrating the ineffectiveness of providing an explicit message rather than a subliminal one.

They Help Quit Smoking

Palmatier, J.R., and Bornstein, P.H. "Effects of Subliminal Stimulation of Symbiotic Merging Fantasies on Behavioral Treatment of Smokers."

The Journal of Nervous and Mental Disease (1980):

- Thirty-four people underwent a package of group therapies to quit smoking for three weeks.

- The results showed that subliminal messages affected the group's behavior after treatment: people who received subliminal messages after regular therapy had a lower percentage of relapse into smoking vice.

A subsequent study by Palmatier and Bornstein showed that 'subliminal messages greatly improved the progress of subjects attempting to quit smoking' compared to the group of people not subjected to subliminal messages.

The Mind Can Hear Subliminal Audio Messages

- The subjects of the experiment listened to a subliminal audio message. The message was mixed with a normal music recording. Another group of subjects simply listened to normal music recordings without subliminal messages.

- Both groups were then asked to create a drawing before the test and immediately after they listened to the music, as well as a drawing of any of the dreams they had had the previous night.

- When the drawings were then examined, you could see the effects of subliminal messages. Drawings of people who listened to music with hidden subliminal messages contained images linked to the suggestions they had been subjected to, while no correlation could be found in the control group.

- Kaser concluded that 'the unconscious/subconscious could perceive a recorded verbal message that cannot be consciously heard, thus proving the existence of subliminal perception.

In another study carried out by Dr. Becker, experimental and control groups were asked to choose a three-digit number. The experimental group had undergone subliminal messages of numbers, inserted into an audio track of "pink noise" (similar to "white noise").

In three different tests, an average of 77% of people subjected to subliminal numbers guessed, as opposed to 10% of the people in the control group. This once again confirms that subliminal messages are perceived at an unconscious level.

Chapter 2.
Losing Weight and Eating Healthily

Silverman and colleagues conducted two subliminal perception experiments with two groups of 26 and 30 women. Women were at least 15% overweight. There were two groups, the "subliminal group" and a "control group."

Both groups were given some education about losing weight and eating healthily, recording calories accurately, having regular mealtimes, and rewarding themselves for eating healthily.

At the beginning and end of all sessions, each was asked to imagine a situation where they might be tempted to overeat.

At this point, they were exposed to a subliminal message for four milliseconds, a subliminal weight loss message for the subliminal group, and a neutral subliminal message for the control group.

In both cases, people belonging to the subliminal group lost more weight than those in the control group, with the subliminal group losing more and more weight towards the end of the treatment period.

It has been concluded that subliminal messages can help people reduce their eating habits too much.

Another study conducted by Dr. Becker showed that the use of subliminal messages could lead to stunning results:

- In Dr. Becker's weight loss clinic at Metairie, Louisiana, her patients listened to music and videotapes containing subliminal messages.

- A woman lost 45 kilos in a year. Subsequently, Dr. Becker found that 50% of patients managed to maintain more than half of the weight loss for the two years following the subliminal message program.

We've seen a lot of stories of people who have been successful at losing weight. You can use subliminal messages to get more success from the efforts you make to lose weight!

Improve Study Skills

Parker, K.A. "Effects of Subliminal Symbiotic Stimulation on Academic Performance: Further Evidence on the Adaptation-Enhancing Effects of Oneness Fantasies." Journal of Counseling Psychology (1982):

- During a summer law school, sixty college students received subliminal messages for six weeks before 3 of their five weekly classes and before and after a one-minute counseling session.

- Subjects exposed to subliminal messages obtained significantly better marks than the others, which turned out to be a constant even in previous studies.

Subliminal Messages to Improve Learning Ability

Cook, H., Ph.D. "Effects of Subliminal Symbiotic Gratification and the Magic of Believing on Achievement." Psychoanalytic Psychology (1985):

- University students were divided into two groups and subjected to either subliminal messages or a control message, immediately after a lesson, for a period of 12 sessions for a subliminal message lasting four milliseconds.

- Students who received subliminal messages performed better at their end-of-year exams than students who received the control message.

- The researchers concluded that subliminally stimulating students to feel better about themselves meant that they studied more profitably.

They Cure Agoraphobia

Lee, I., Tyrer, P. and Horn, S., "A comparison of Subliminal, Supraliminal and Faded Phobic Cine-Films in the Treatment of Agoraphobia." British Journal of Psychiatry (1983):

- Thirty-two patients were treated for two-week videos over two weeks. Three of the groups saw the same film—a selection of agoraphobia scenes, while the control group saw a potter working on his lathe. The three groups tested included a group that saw the images at a level below the view threshold (subliminal group), one that saw it under normal conditions (regular group), and a third that was subjected to both subliminal and regular vision as the study progressed (faded group).

- The faded group was the one that showed the greatest improvements compared to the other groups. The improvement also lasted for twelve weeks.

- These results indicate that the presentation of both subliminal and regular messages can reduce agoraphobic behaviors, but there is a much greater effect when combined.

Precision in Darts Play

Plumbo, R. and Gillman, I. "Effects of Subliminal Activation of Oedipal Fantasies on Competitive Performance." 1984: The Journal of Nervous and Mental Disease.

- Subjects have been tested for their accuracy in darts play. They were exposed to the following subliminal messages: "Beating my opponent is a good thing," "Beating my opponent is a bad thing, and a neutral message of control: "People walk. "

- The results show that people subjected to the message "Beating my opponent is a good thing" showed better accuracy at the darts game than those who had heard another message.

This study shows that even a simple positive message I transmit while playing darts can lead to a better accuracy level.

Strong Reactions to Subconscious Messages

Bornstein, R.F, Leone, D.R. and Galley, D.J. "The Generalizability of Subliminal Mere Exposure Effects: Influence of Stimuli Perceived Without Awareness on Social Behavior." Journal of Personality and Social Psychology (1987):

- The subjects tested have been made to hear hidden statements from "white noise" to an ever-increasing volume.

- Strong psychological reactions were observed in subjects exposed to messages masquerading as a strong "white noise" and, therefore, inaudible, rather than when the volume was lower. The messages could be somewhat audible.

- Research has concluded that completely inaudible messages could reach the human mind and have a psychological effect.

Subliminal Messages Reduce Shoplifting

- TIME Magazine reported in 1979 that nearly 50 department stores in the United States and Canada used subliminal messages in their music playback systems, reducing both shopliftings by customers and employee theft.

- An East Coast chain has come to save $600,000 over nine months!

- Another story told in the Wall Street Journal in 1980 led to the claim that subliminal messages in a New Orleans supermarket resulted in a significant reduction in theft, from $50,000 in six months to $13,000!

Also, cash drops fell from $125 a week to $10 a week.

The Power of Subliminal Stimulus

Shevrin, H. "Does the Averaged Evoked Response Encode Subliminal Perception? Yes." (1975):

- These studies have shown that different people's responses to a provided stimulus are statistically lower when subjects are consciously aware of receiving it. Still, when the stimulus was administered subliminally, the response rate was significantly higher.

- Although people were unaware of the stimuli they were getting, the measurements suggest that our minds are aware of it instead. This indicates that while our mind is not consciously aware of a message, our subconscious can take a subliminal message on board and respond as if it were transposed under normal conditions.

If you want more information about subliminal messages, you can check our How Subliminal Messages work page or our FAQs on subliminal messages. If you have any further questions, you can contact us directly.

Our subliminal suggestions are mainly positive statements, which will penetrate your mind subliminally, without distracting you and without being aware of them.

The main advantage of using an audio or video subliminal album is that you can save time—you don't have to stand in front of the mirror every morning and evening and repeat the claims to yourself. It's an effortless method—you can also play while listening to the album and doing many other things, working, studying, exercising. You can also learn subliminal messages while you sleep. Check out our Subliminal Catalog—you'll find a wide range of over 200 titles; no matter what you're looking for, you'll surely find something that matches your needs.

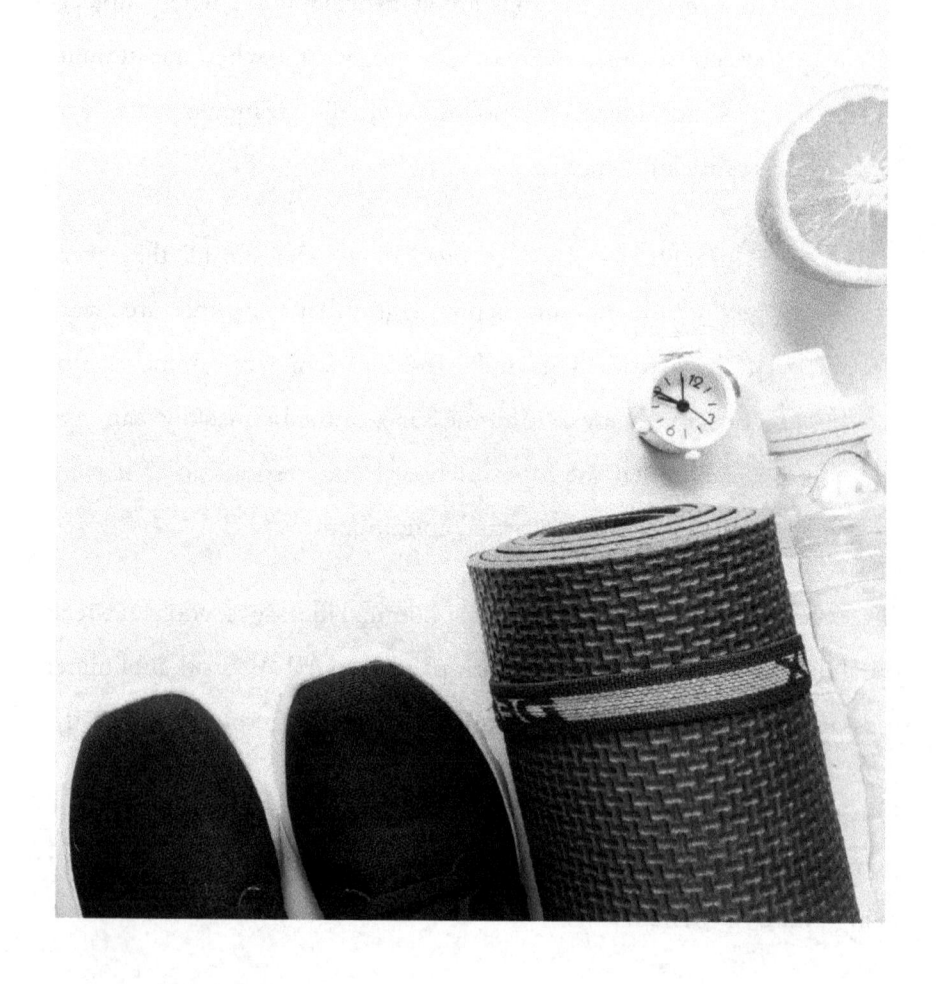

Chapter 3.
Identify New Ways to Cope With Stress

Each of us experiences various stress levels; we have to manage stress at work, for issues that arise by administering and developing a business, or for personal situations that sometimes overwhelm us.

Stress is one of those things that, if not addressed, tend to generate additional problems. It can affect sleep, decreasing our performance; if we do not find a way to manage stress, the situation can worsen.

Simply observing how negative stress is would be too trivial and simplistic. Our relationship with stress is much more complex: the point is not just to know how to overcome it; it is also about knowing how to understand and manage stress, exploiting it to become more productive.

The Causes of Stress

According to psychologist Walter Cannon, creator of the concept known as the "attack or escape "reaction, the primary function of stress would be to allow survival.

Stress is often a useful reaction to challenges or threats: it makes us mentally and physically ready to face them. It chemically affects our brain, raising the level of attention, intensifying cognitive activity, and increasing sensory abilities.

But in other circumstances, where it has no practical purpose or persists longer than necessary, it can be harmful and have negative consequences. Ultimately, stress is how we react to stressors: real or just perceived challenges—to address real or only perceived needs.

Stressors, called stressors, may have an inner or external origin:

- **External stressors:** These are environmental or work changes, new or difficult tasks to perform, events totally beyond our control, such as deadlines, a thunderstorm, or the accounts to be paid.

- **Internal stressors:** Normally, thoughts or behaviors, sleep or eat badly, or feelings of anger or anxiety.

However, not all types of stress are the same. A distinction must be made between acute and chronic stress.

Acute Stress Gives Us "Superpowers"

We all know this kind of stress. It makes us awake and responsive in the moment of the challenges or emotions of the day. It can help us if there is an actual threat with real consequences (e.g., an important deadline).

If you are a serial procrastinator, there is a good chance that you will only give your best if you have a high level of acute stress, so, normally, close to a deadline. Deadlines would be just a positive stressor looking at things from this perspective, useful to increase productivity.

However, acute episodic or frequent stress, very common for those leading chaotic lives, can overexcite the mind, which is confusing, counterproductive, and can lead to a nervous breakdown.

Chronic Stress Harms the Quality of Our Lives

It's what we usually call "bad stress"; it wears us down over time. It is often the result of persistent environmental conditions: a job we do not like, an unsealed relationship, or economic difficulties.

Chronic stress can affect sleep quality and, in fact, accelerate the aging process. We can't always avoid the sources of chronic stress in our lives. But, at least to some extent, we can control and manage stress.

Eustress and Distress

Stress Is Not Necessarily Negative

Some people are productive under stress and need to stay under pressure to be more operational. On the other hand, other meticulously plan everything to avoid having to manage stress, at least as long as possible. There is no fair and wrong kind of approach. It's just important to be aware of how you react to stress, giving due weight to the duties you face.

Eustress is the right amount of stress, which helps us to increase our productivity; Moreover, in the absence of total stress, some tasks would be difficult to tackle with due care.

Distress, or excessive stress, can be a source of agitation and bring frustration, anxiety, depression, poor performance, and other negative consequences.

According to Yerkes-Dodson's slaw, to perform work that requires resistance (routine and tedious, or long tasks to complete), one could benefit from higher levels of acute stress.

Simultaneously, one could normally concentrate better on new tasks in the absence of excessive pressure.

How to Manage Stress in 6 Strategies

We've seen what stressors are and how they can affect our lives. Now let's look at some strategies to manage stress most effectively.

Probably, the following will encourage us to change the way we see things and beyond. It will also help us change the way we spend our most precious resource: time.

Give Priority to What Is Important and Not to What Is Urgent

It is often difficult between work and family to avoid having an infinite number of things to do. It is difficult to determine where to start; every task seems to have the same importance. That is why it is essential to manage stress, to have a reliable criterion that allows us to distribute our workload according to priorities.

It can be easy to assign priorities to tasks based on their simplicity or their brevity. But a popular method is to evaluate each fulfillment based on two criteria:

- **Importance:** Does completing the task contribute to the achievement of your professional and personal objectives?

- **Urgency:** The task must be completed soon. Otherwise, will there be negative consequences?

Stress Can Be Managed

The word stress has now fully entered the common language with numerous meanings and sometimes in contrast to each other (tension, anxiety, fatigue, apprehension, depression, illness, etc.). To work together on this theme, the first step necessary for the maintenance of mental health, we propose a definition of stress to be shared and from which to start: it is the set of changes/reactions in physical, mental, or behavioral functioning that are activated in the individual in response to a request for adaptation concerning new biological, environmental or psychological-relational needs.

It is a neutral concept, a "normal" response that has allowed the species' evolution.

That becomes negative only when the stimuli continue over time or exceed the resources available to cope with it. In this case, we are talking about distress, as opposed to eustress (positive).

We suggest the following three steps to address the broad theme of stress management successfully:

- Know (stressors)
- Recognize (stress reactions)
- Manage (strategies)

Knowing Stress

Stressors that during service and mission periods could generate an "accumulation" of stress are of two types: physical and mental. Learning to identify which of these concern us at certain times in our personal and working lives and the "weight" they have for each of us is the first step in preparing ourselves to face them effectively.

Physical Stressors

Environmental

- Hot, cold, humidity

- Vibrations, harassing noises, explosions

- Intense lights, poor visibility, darkness

- Fumes, particulates

- Chemical agents, infectious agents, ionizing radiation

- Rough, muddy, dusty terrain

- Nauseating smells

Physiological

- Sleep deprivation

- Dehydration

- Malnutrition

- Muscle/aerobic fatigue

- Poor hygiene conditions

- Depressed immune system

- Injuries, injuries, pathologies, trauma

Mental Stressors

Cognitive

- Information problems (deficient, excessive, ambiguous, changeable)

- Decision-making problems

- Role uncertainty

- Unpredictability of events

- Restructuring of its value system

- Imperfect organizational dynamics

Emotional and Social

- Threats that induce fear, anxiety, terror

- The occurrence of critical events

- Idle boredness

- Isolation or inaccessibility of social support

- Conflict with colleagues/superiors/family members

Recognize

Stress reactions (signs of discomfort) and everyone's perception of stressful stimuli are extremely variable and depend on aspects of personality and experience.

There are, however, some reactions that can be defined as common and that manifest themselves in different areas of our operation. Learning to recognize these signals early allows us to understand their causes, give them meaning, and begin to act.

Manage

There may be many strategies to be put in place to deal with stress and the first signs of discomfort when they arise.

They depend on our personal coping styles, the availability of the context we find ourselves, and how personal, relational, and professional individual functioning is limited by discomfort.

Identifying what we can do to manage negative stress is a fundamental step to act and become aware of the actions that can help recover our psychophysical balance.

Your Coping Style

Coping is the set of cognitive and coping strategies centered on emotions: they express their emotions by talking to friends and other significant people, adapting emotionally to the problematic situation. In this way, it is often possible to recognize one's emotional state and manage it properly. Behavioral conditions that an individual puts in place to manage and deal with stressful situations. You can classify coping styles into three types:

- **Task-centered coping:** The task we focus on is the solution to the problem, often sought directly and immediately. When the problem is easy to solve, this type is effective and economical. Otherwise, this strategy is dysfunctional.

- **Emotion-centered coping:** They express their emotions by talking to friends and other significant people, adapting emotionally to the problematic situation. In this way, it is often possible to recognize one's emotional state and manage it properly.

- **Coping centered on avoidance:** Contact with the stressor is avoided; the source of stress is not eliminated, but the individual is distracted by the cognitive perception of the stressor. Such a strategy is effective in the short term, to take an emotional break from an emotionally charged situation, which does not present large margins of the solution in the immediate future.

You should know that there are no right or wrong coping styles because strategies that can be effective in one situation may not be effective.

Effective reactive modes themselves can become negative if used exclusively. Especially in stressful events lasting over time, it is important to not tighten up on a single strategy but to change it if it proves ineffective and deactivated.

Some Actions That Work to Prevent and Manage Stress

- **Do physical activity:** It is a certain fact that exercise is one of the best stress-reduction techniques.

- **Sleep well:** Give yourself due hours of sleep/rest.

- **Follow a balanced diet:** Keep a healthy and correct diet.

- **Count your alcohol, tobacco, and coffee intake:** The use of these substances increases stress rather than reducing it!

- **Take it easy:** Allow yourself free time to do what you like: reading, music, writing, drawing.

- **Manage your time better:** Set priorities and, as far as the assignment allows you, create effective work/rest rhythms.

- **Humor:** Laughing helps reduce tension.

- **Recognize your emotions:** It is normal to feel angry or upset. Feelings are natural reactions to stressful circumstances.

- **Talk to someone you trust:** Use colleagues and friends as a sounding board, often just vent to get better. Other times, they can help you find a solution.

- **Accept reality:** Only a few things can be influenced and changed. Invest your energy in these, not situations out of your control. Learn to be open-minded and flexible; it will help you adapt more effectively.

When all this is not enough, and the discomfort persists, you can think of turning to a specialist who can help you understand the malaise's reasons and find the right way to manage it and recover your balance!

How to Fight Stress

"Stress" is the evolutionarily determined response to internal or external factors that require immediate intervention by the body. The state of stress mobilizes a large amount of energy to improve performance for a short period. Such activation is usually reduced when the causes are removed, and the organism can quickly re-enter a state of normality.

In contemporary societies, however, it often happens that the environment's demands remain for a long time. This goes far beyond our body's ability to sustain a stressful situation, for example, a state of economic poverty, too long working hours, demand-studded working days, family problems, or chronic diseases. In these and many other cases, the stress response is not disabled, leading to resource depletion and side effects called "metabolic syndrome." Also, it has been shown that the condition of chronic stress leads to habituation such that the person begins to get used to and lose awareness of the physical and social symptoms that characterize it.

The most common signs of the stress response are:

- Presence of emotions such as anger, irritability, anxiety, and depression

- Musculoskeletal pain such as migraine, pain in the back, jaw, neck

- Digestive problems such as stomach acidity, gastroesophageal reflux, diarrhea, constipation, and irritable colon syndrome

- Increased blood pressure, acceleration of heart rate, sweating, tremors, shortness of breath, or a sense of chest oppression

Here, then, it becomes necessary to find useful strategies to reduce physiological activation and combat stress.

Awareness

The first step is to monitor the signals that the mind and body show when under stress. Every person experiences this state differently, and, therefore, it is necessary to ask: "what do I think? How do I feel, and what sensations do I have when I'm under stress?" For example, some people have difficulty concentrating; others feel irritable and furious; others still experience tiredness and poor appetite.

Stress is a non-specific response, activated by any situation perceived as superior to its forces. It is, therefore, important to identify the daily events that lead to activate the stress response. Do they have anything to do with the family? The job? The care of the house?

Defining and taking note of these situations helps combat stress and prevent and manage its side effects. Once you can recognize the stress signals and the situations that activate them, managing the stress response's physiological activation is necessary.

Dealing With Stress

A second strategy is to take a step back from these situations and permit yourself to take a break. Dedicating yourself to something that reduces the state of stress can only improve the way you deal with it. Some of these activities are presented below.

Exercise

Much research has now shown that exercise has a powerful anti-stress effect. When addressed regularly, the exercise produces substances called endorphins. These counteract unpleasant feelings of stress and produce a feeling of energy and vitality. The literature shows that even 20 minutes of walking a day can be beneficial for many hours.

Diaphragm Respiration

The rhythm and type of breathing can greatly impact the physiological aspects of the stressful state. In general, two types of breathing can be distinguished. The high or clavicular one involving the chest muscles and the lower or diaphragm muscles that use the diaphragm (the dome muscle used precisely for breathing) is greater.

Usually, in times of high stress due to muscle tension, people mainly use the first breathing type. In doing so, however, they fill the lungs less and increase the respiratory rhythm. On the contrary, diaphragm respiration has a slower and more constant rhythm. This type of breathing can greatly reduce the physiological activation of the organism.

It can be useful to lie on a bed and rest your hands on the belly to learn this breathing. If during inhalation, it swells, then the breathing is the diaphragm. Otherwise, you will have to try, very kindly, to inflate it with each inhales. It is useful to emphasize how you should not strive to "throw out" the belly. It is enough to relax the abdominal muscles to make room for the contraction of the diaphragm.

Once you have learned this type of breathing, valid to combat stress, you can do short sessions of ten minutes a day. The inhale must last for about three seconds, while the suction should last for five seconds. Lengthening the time of air escaping from the lungs naturally stimulates our relaxation response through the vagus nerve.

Meditation

The literature indicates that daily practicing a form of meditation reduces psychological and physical tension. Therefore, it is not surprising that one of the most effective protocols for stress management is Mindfulness-Based Stress Reduction.

It is based on mindfulness meditation, which aims to develop a new way of relating to one's thoughts and emotions.

Relaxation Techniques

Relaxation is the psychophysiological state in which the activity of the body stabilizes at levels of normality. When in this state, the physicist is not solicited to respond to environmental requests and therefore is perceived as a state of well-being and serenity.

To reduce stress, especially if chronic, it can be useful to learn relaxation techniques. The most widespread and historically effective procedure is Jacobson's progressive muscle relaxation. It involves alternating moments when some muscles are voluntarily contracted and moments when these muscles are released.

For example, you can start shaking hands for five seconds and then suddenly release them for the next fifteen. You will then move on to your arms, shoulders, thighs, feet, face, and then start the cycle again and complete it three times.

If the exercise is done daily, it will become easier and easier to recall the state of relaxation in a few weeks, allowing you to enter even thinking of relaxing.

Sleep Hygiene

An often underestimated aspect of the strategy to combat stress symptoms is respect for the amount and quality of sleep humans need. When we are under stress, the hormones responsible for physiological activation (glucocorticoids) stimulate the brain by making it difficult to fall asleep or disturb the deep sleep stages. At the same time, sleep is when the brain recharges with energy; deprivation of hours of rest leads to memory difficulties and concentration during wakefulness. These are themselves a source of stress.

That's why curing sleep hygiene is critical to reducing stress. The main precautions are:

- Ensure at least seven hours of sleep per night.
- Build yourself a sleep routine before bedtime, for example, always doing the same things in the ten minutes before bed.

- Eat lightly in the evening so that you are not yet in the digestive phase when bedtime.

- Engage in relaxing activities in the ninety minutes before bed.

- Confine the intake of stimulants such as coffee, tea, chocolate, or nicotine in the morning and never before bed.

- Ensure an adequate environment for rest, therefore good air quality and a temperature around eighteen degrees.

Maintaining Social Relationships

Frequently what happens when requests, especially the work increase, is the reduction of social and leisure activities; this, if understandable, has harmful effects on psychological and physical well-being. Having moments of sharing with loved ones has a powerful anti-stress effect on the human organism. The connection with others regulates the emotional state and allows the organism to rebalance.

How to Manage Stress Through the Act

Know how to manage stress. In the face of particularly challenging periods in our lives, we can experience chronic fatigue managing stress. In other cases, particularly serious events can happen that lead us to exclaim, "It's as if the world has collapsed on me!" In the face of intense or unexpected periods, unwanted changes, bereavements, illnesses, emotionally stressful situations, it is possible to feel a sense of heaviness, fear, blocking. It is appropriate to learn how to manage stress, to recognize how our mind works automatically, and discover new ways to govern our internal emotional states.

How to Manage Stress

It is important to learn how to manage stress practically. We often face stressful moments by discussing motivational behaviors (we eat more, smoke, excel in alcoholic substances, etc.). "Any pressure or request that comes from the environment can trigger a stress response." Says Dr. Nicola Maffini, psychologist and psychotherapist.

"But what makes the difference in our lives and for our well-being is the way we perceive and manage those events." "Learning to manage stress, therefore, becomes fundamental.

Certain events are more stressful, such as the loss of a loved one, the sudden loss of work, the discovery of a serious illness, but in most cases, it is how we report to these events that determines how much stress they cause us".

"There are people," says Dr. Maffini, "who may realize that they have difficulty managing small or large unexpected events, who often feel crushed by difficulties, and who feel trapped in trying to fight even small changes." It is possible that these people, failing to manage stress, face problems such as anxiety, depression, difficulty in sleep, organic pathologies of varying severity. Therefore, it is important to become aware of these difficulties and understand how to manage these moments in the best way to experience stressful events less oppressively and more healthily.

How to Manage Stress According to the ACT

"Experiencing stressful events or dealing with particularly painful situations is part of the life of each of us," continues Dr. Maffini, "and according to the ACT, we call this clean pain." Clean pain is the stress that everyone experiences in the face of a difficult event. She is sad in the face of mourning, worried about a sudden change, fatigued by an illness. "To experience these feelings in the face of the adversity of life is normal."

When we try not to feel this stress, trying to anesthetize it, then the problems begin. Our ways of anesthetizing ourselves, in the long run, don't work. Indeed feed suffering on suffering. Let's take an example if to manage the stress of daily life (and the anxieties related to this) I use, for example, alcohol, I might notice after a short period that anesthetizing that stress by drinking in the long term does not work. It worsens my state of health, increasing my stress.

"This worsening of initial stress, in the ACT, we call it dirty pain. What is dirty pain? Dirty pain is all that more pain that we create, so we don't feel clean pain." Therefore, learning to manage stress means opening up to body sensations, even unpleasant related to stress, and starting to listen to each other.

Our mind can absorb and elaborate adaptive responses to a stressful event. But our behaviors may not help this process. If we are stressed, we do everything to "not feel" the pain, worry, and tiredness, then we risk blocking these adaptive processes of the mind.

Managing Stress Through Mindfulness

A good and effective practice to open up to the sensations of one's body and observe the natural functioning of the mind is mindfulness. Mindfulness, an oriental meditative practice, is particularly effective in stress management and other psychological distress situations.

"Managing stress (whatever the cause) requires, first of all, abandoning all those automatic behaviors that we use to anesthetize ourselves. And mindfulness is a powerful ally in this. Through practice, it is possible to "observe" in a non-judgmental and welcoming way one's reactions to stress, not by "putting them under the carpet."

Mindfulness Center of the Maria Luigia Hospital conducts mindfulness meditations open to everyone every week. Also, group courses for stress management are organized regularly. For more information on all the routes organized at the Maria Luigia Hospital clinic, you can visit the page of the Courses of their mindfulness center.

Fighting Stress Causes Symptoms and Remedies

In industrialized societies, stress is increasingly being heard. Understanding what causes stress, identifying all the symptoms of stress, and finding the "cure for stress" are just some of the issues that we look for daily. Stress is a strategic response that the organism uses to adapt to any external pressure that alters its balance. If the stress reaction is prolonged over time, we talk about chronic stress.

The real enemy, therefore, would not be individual acute stress events (such as a dispute with the boss at work or a discussion with the partner), but stressful life situations that continue over time (for example, hostile work environment, bereave affairs, chronic diseases of their own or a relative).

Let's find out together how to combat chronic stress, starting with its causes and its main symptoms.

Sources of Stress

What causes stress? In an attempt to figure out how to combat psychophysical stress, all of us have asked ourselves this question at least once in our lives. It is not possible to identify a unique cause, so let's group main ideas about the origin of stress into three macro-categories:

- Environment

- Personal answers

- The transaction between individual and environment

When you only consider the environmental causes, you often hear about work stress, competition stress, marriage stress, study stress, stress caused by children's growth, etc.

The necessary restrictions to which we have all had to adapt, together with the fear of contagion, can be a big stress source, especially in the long term. For this reason, the Order of Psychologists suggests 20 rules to be adopted to develop resilience and promote collective well-being.

Other theories about the origin of stress consider the individual response to counter the event that threatens one's state of well-being. The response to combat psychophysical stress involves physiological, emotional, cognitive, and behavioral reactions.

According to the most accredited scientific explanations, we are not just victims of stressful events.

To cause stress and fatigue (physical and mental), we jointly intervene in the way we evaluate the events that happen to us, the resources that we can identify in ourselves and the environment, and the evaluation of our ability to use them effectively to eradicate the threat.

Regarding to the stress symptoms, where does all that tension go? How do we understand when we're stressed? One of the first sensations we feel when we are under stress is the state of tension, both physical and mental. This is due to the perception that the environment's demands are greater than the resources and strategies we normally use to cope with them.

When we are faced with persistent and severe stress, what causes in us? Let's see what the physical and psychological consequences of stress are.

Researchers at the Canadian Institute of Stress have defined five phases, which correspond to as many classes of symptoms of chronic distress:

- **Chronic fatigue (physical or mental):** it can manifest itself with difficulty falling asleep, often accompanied by unhealthy habits in an attempt to relax (such as smoking or drinking alcohol). It is difficult to get out of bed in the morning, and during the day, you look for caffeine or other exciting substances. Symptoms of mental stress also include difficulty concentrating and memory.

- **Interpersonal problems and self-isolation:** relationship difficulties, such as family conflicts and problems at work, increase. The mental fatigue and physical discomfort that goes hand in hand with chronic stress experience can wear down our relationships, gradually leading to isolation. In this way, everyday problems can also appear as insurmountable rocks.

- **Emotional turbulence:** The tendency to isolation increases and the lack of perceived social support makes it difficult to manage time and identify priorities. Frequent mood swings accompany stress and mental confusion, and difficulty regulating emotions, making us feel insecure, unable to make choices and make decisions.

- **Chronic pain:** The first physical symptom is muscle tension, especially in the neck, shoulders, lower back, and face. At night frequently, you tend to tighten the jaws by grinding your teeth (bruxism) as if to discharge the tension. Common is the so-called "weekend" headaches, resulting from the sudden return of normal flow to the head's blood vessels after days of forced compression.

- **Stress disorders:** At this stage, the symptoms of chronic stress result in real pathologies (see Table 1), resulting from a progressive weakening of the immune system.

Fight stress with some remedies. In the face of stressful events, the primary response that each of us puts in place can be summarized in the expression "fight or flight," attack, or flight.

Attention, not always directly addressing what threatens our well-being, is the most appropriate solution.

Sometimes you need to get distracted, take time, and find out before finding the most suitable facing strategy for the situation.

Below we suggest a series of remedies to combat stress.

Eliminate Daily Stress on 10 Tips

How many times have you wondered, "how to overcome stress?". Among the remedies that can be used to relieve stress, there are many strategies that each of us can use independently and that does not require the possession of particular skills.

These ten tips will help you understand how to treat stress naturally.

Foods to Combat Stress

Proper nutrition is essential to increase immune defenses and combat oxidative stress.

In dealing with prolonged stress, some nutrients are necessary for our organism (such as vitamin B, vitamin C, zinc, and magnesium) to run out more quickly.

it is useful to replenish the necessary vitamins to combat stress, opt for a diet that is as varied as possible, and that includes:

- Carbohydrates (better if whole grains)
- Vegetables (species of green color)
- Fresh and dried fruit
- Legumes

What are the foods that fight stress, and that contains nutrients that should never be missed? Before making some examples of foods to combat stress, a premise, no food in itself, effectively combats stress when taken in a climate of tension. As a general rule, it is advisable to choose light meals to consume calmly, in a comfortable environment.

- **Citrus:** Oranges, lemons, mandarins, and grapefruits are recommended because they are rich in vitamin C and flavonoids; these foods are a powerful ally to fight infections, lower blood pressure and cortisol levels in the blood.

- **Green tea:** A steaming cup of green tea or a warm herbal tea helps keep cellular hydration high, necessary for muscles and joints' optimal functioning. Amino acid theanine, contained in tea, promotes lowering blood pressure in adult subjects. If you've wondered how to dispose of the nervousness of a hectic day, you might try to indulge in a cup of hot tea every night.

- **Milk:** A cup of hot milk is one of the most common natural remedies to combat stress and nervousness. The calcium in milk helps to feel more energetic and improves the mood tone, thanks to phospholipids' contribution. To learn more about cow's milk's effects on human health, we recommend reading the Nutrition Foundation of Italy's document.

- **Dried fruits:** Nuts, almonds, pistachios, and all dried fruits are typically rich in vitamin E, magnesium, fiber, and good fats, useful to improve stress reactivity. The recommended dose of dried fruit for an average adult, as indicated by the Italian Society of Human Nutrition, is 30g per day.

- **Tuna salmon and sardines:** Salmon contains omega three and helps fight the inflammatory state that is a consequence of stress; the bluefish (cod, mackerel, sardines), on the other hand, is rich in vitamin D3, which stimulates the immune system, reduces inflammation, and prevents infections. The Italian Ministry of Health recommends consuming fish 2-3 times a week.

Reduce Stress With a Hot Bath

During a hot bath, the heat experienced facilitates muscles' relaxation, favoring a consequent increase in mental relaxation. Other beneficial effects are the improvement of blood circulation and the feeling of increased energy.

How to Decrease Stress With a Pet

Research from Washington State University helps us figure out how to combat study stress. According to experts, it takes 10 minutes a day of direct interaction with a pet, such as a dog or a cat. Playing or cuddling these animals combated school stress effectively, reducing students' cortisol levels significantly (known as the "stress hormone").

Our four-legged friends also help counteract stress fatigue in the workplace.

According to a study published in the journal "International Journal of Workplace Health Management," bringing your dog to the office reduces work stress and improves employee concentration and productivity.

How to Overcome Stress by Spending Time Outdoors

A way to slow down and take a break from the hectic pace of daily life can be found in spending time outdoors, such as taking walks to the sea or hiking in the mountains. Even the choice to live in a maritime resort, rather than in a city house, can make a difference: living by the sea makes you happy!

One of the activities to practice outside, even when you only have a balcony at your disposal, is gardening. Moving pots and handling shovels, rakes, and shears helps keep your mind busy and focused on the present, driving away concerns about future events or past-related displeasure.

Exposure to sunlight also stimulates vitamin D production, essential for producing endorphins such as serotonin and dopamine, which help improve mood tone.

How to Drain Stress With Art

Painting, drawing, coloring, shaping a ceramic, sewing a dress, playing, or doing theater: each of these activities has proven effective in combating stress naturally. It is no coincidence that we are talking about art therapy. Creating and expressing oneself leads people to feel good and relieve the symptoms of chronic stress. Let's find out why, with the help of some examples.

How to Combat Psychological Stress

Mandalas can be the ideal solution to combat nervousness and stress. Engaging in an activity that requires moderate cognitive concentration and manual work such as coloring a complex and elaborate design – allows anyone to lighten their mind from everyday life worries.

The consequent benefits of relaxation and mental relaxation will also be reflected in the body.

How to Reduce Stress With Music

Music is a natural antistress accessible to everyone. Listening to relaxing music to combat stress or even singing or playing an instrument can be ideal solutions. Fighting chronic stress with music allows you to loosen tension, driving away bad thoughts and increasing brain production of substances such as endorphin, which function as natural analgesics improving mood.

How to Get Rid of Stress With Writing

Since the studies of James Pennebaker, creator of the expressive writing technique, the role of writing as a tool to relieve stress has been widely recognized.

Writing has been shown to help reduce mental and physical stress, linked to different types of potentially destabilizing events for the person (pregnancy management, breakdown of a relationship, loss of work, stress for university exams, etc.). Writing helps clarify and explain what causes stress, favoring the use of effective facing strategies.

Reduce Stress With Sexual Activity

For some people, especially when stress is not excessive, sexual activity can relieve the tension accumulated during the week and combat the physical consequences of stress. For example, who has not had difficulty falling asleep after a day full of commitments and worries?

How to Manage Stress With Humor

Humor turned out to be a great strategy to prevent and manage stress. For example, in healthcare, clown therapy has now spread, made famous by the story of Patch Adams, and told by the film of the same name starring Robin Williams. Patch Adams teaches us that self-irony can turn into natural medicine, at no cost, to combat stress and depression.

How to Relieve Stress With Prosociality

Numerous studies have observed that prosocial behavior can be a relevant factor in preserving one's well-being in stressful living conditions, such as comparing with traumatic experiences.

Focusing our thinking on helping someone else, rather than their fears, is a cure-all for reducing anxiety.

Fighting Stress With Sport

Practicing sports to vent stress is useful, as long as physical activity is not experienced as an obligation but as something pleasant and fun. There is no advantage in doing sports if this causes even more stress or pressure for the competition. There are no specific exercises to combat stress, but an activity best suits the person's needs.

Some may prefer to engage in aerobic activities such as running and team sports that promote socialization. Among the latter, the WAL (Walk and Learn) method has proved effective in reducing symptoms of anxiety, stress, and depression. Exercise produces biochemical changes that improve mental health. An example of this is the increase in endorphin levels in the brain, morphine-like substances that produce an immediate well-being feeling. The WHO recommends practicing physical activity for at least 3 hours a week. Knowing some exercises to do at home could be useful never to have to give up physical activity.

How a Professional Can Help You Fight Stress

"Despite all the efforts and efforts, I keep feeling stressed": do you wonder how to eliminate stress? To combat psychophysical stress, "natural" remedies and self-help strategies that we have described so far are not always enough. In some cases, requesting a professional's help, such as a psychologist or a doctor, can be the smartest choice to make. Thanks to these professionals' support, you can strengthen your resources and learn new remedies for stress to regain your well-being.

Relaxation Techniques

The relaxation techniques useful to relieve mental and physical stress are numerous, and some of them can be learned with extreme ease and at any age. The learning of these techniques has no contraindications. We can all benefit from them by applying them to the most varied types of potentially stressful situations. Among the most common relaxation techniques, we mention Diaphragm Breathing, Progressive Muscle Relaxation, and Biofeedback.

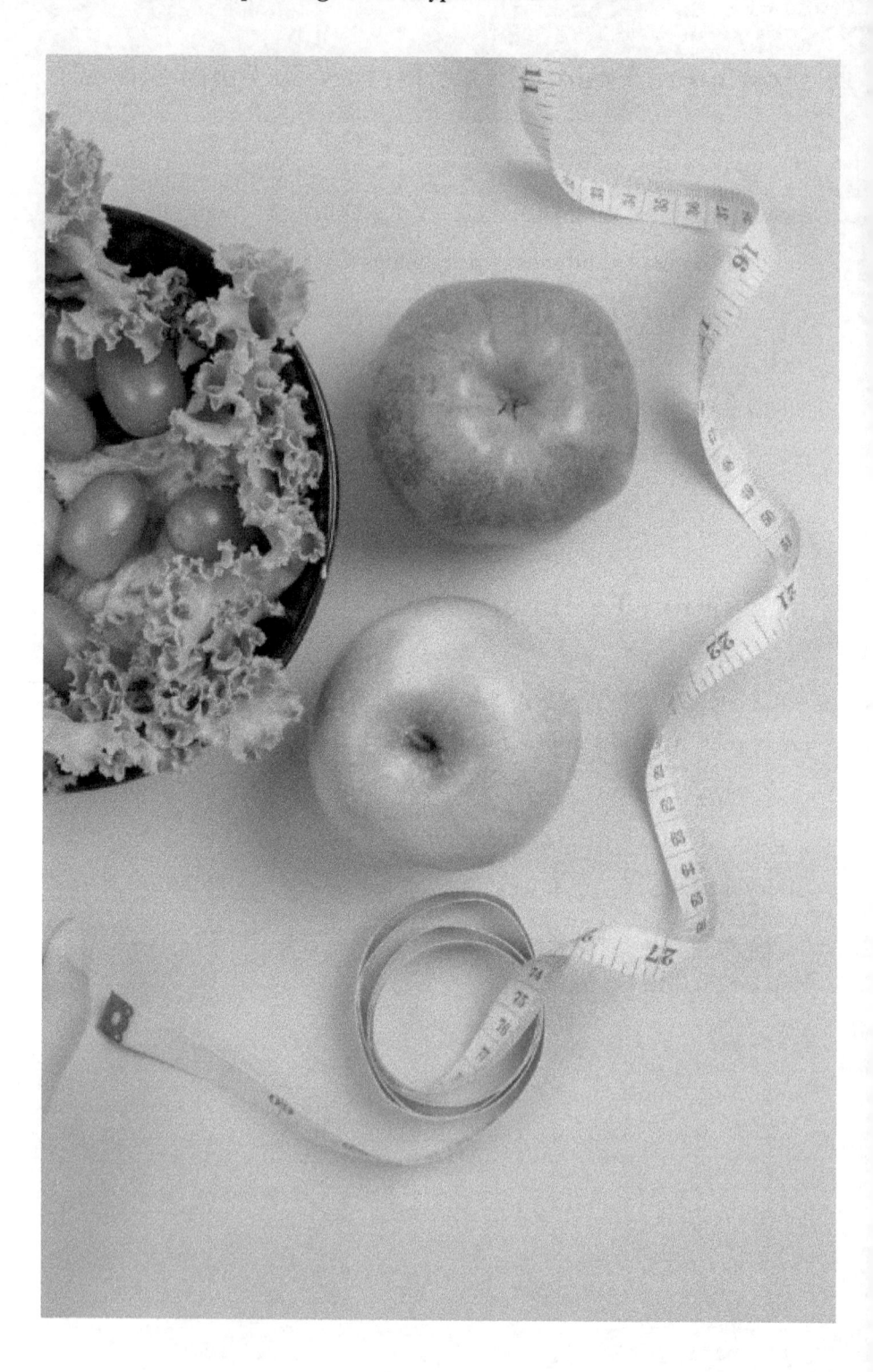

Chapter 4.
Get Back on Track

The holiday season is often seen as the proverbial ground zero for out-of-control food choices, choices that effectively ruin all the hard work you've done in the gym and kitchen in previous months. But while none of us here at HealthSPORT recommends going completely off the rails with the diet (who wants to feel swollen and icky?), we recommend people remember that your healthy lifestyle is just that: A LIFESTYLE.

And guess what? Lifestyles have natural flows and flow towards them. No one should feel obliged to follow a strict, clean, and 100% no-frills diet and do a physical activity all the time, especially during the holidays, which are full of homemade delicacies, family traditions, and convivial meetings.

Seriously, life is not so strict, so why should you be? That said, we understand if you're a little worried about figuring out how to enjoy a guilt-free vacation without going completely out to sea in decadent sauces and desserts.

To that end, we're preparing a few things to think about as you prepare for the upcoming Thanksgiving (or Friendsgiving) so you can go back from the "day off" with aplomb and a lot of turkey leftover.

Don't Bite Any More Than You Can Chew

On the day or two after Thanksgiving, you may be tempted to make a pencil in a ton of training sessions, training classes, and meal preparation days to "catch up" whatever you've decided to indulge in on the big day. The problem with trying to go from 0 to 60 is that you can easily overwhelm yourself and cause a serious flare-up. That is, your high schedule is unreasonable, so instead of downsizing it, you give up and slip back into those Thanksgiving pants at Friends' Joey Tribbiani (Christmas will come soon, anyway, right?).

If you're looking to get back to a diet and post-T Day exercise routine, be realistic. Increase the intensity and frequency, and try not to raise your eyes so high that you completely lose focus.

Concrete Extract

Setting a goal between Thanksgiving and the end of the year can be a great way to keep you motivated and excited about your workouts (as if you weren't already!). But instead of something as vague as "I'll train more from now on" or "I'll eat clean until Christmas," stick to a more specific goal that you can answer "yes" or "no" if you're asked, "Did you get this?" Examples of concrete examples could be:

- I'm going to the gym three times a week.

- I'm not going to drink soda.

- I'm going to incorporate some vegetables into every meal.

Again, be reasonable, but remember the classic adage about management: if you can't measure it, you can't handle it.

Become a Self-Care Expert

No matter where you are on your journey with fitness and health, holidays can elicit a lot of guilt. I shouldn't eat it. I should be able to stay clean. I should, and I should. Listen: no one has achieved greatness by being mean to himself. So, during the holiday season, commit to acting self-decomposing every day, or at least a couple of times a week. Give yourself a hand/Pedi, drink plenty of water, write in a diary, watch funny movies (hi Elf!). Doing what you think makes you feel loved, appreciated, and grateful.

What to fill you with inspiration in this holiday season? Today, contact the HealthSPORT team to learn about personal training, group fitness classes, 10-day passes, and all the other services we offer in Humboldt County.

6 Ways to Stabilize Weight Loss

It is a situation where most people on a low-carb diet can identify with: after a period of progressive weight loss, they suddenly hit a plateau and can no longer lose the kilos too much as they did before. Alternatively, you may follow a maintenance diet, and after stepping on the bathroom ladder, find that you fired a couple of pounds.

While there may be some physiological explanations for this, particularly in the early stages of a diet, it may also be due to certain bad habits that have crept in or the steps in your weight loss program that you failed to take.

The first thing to do is not panic. The weight fluctuates; it happens to all of us.

However, if a month goes by and your weight is still fluctuating or completely stalled, there are a few steps you can take to get back on track.

Avoid Carb Creep

Even a busy diet can sometimes get carbohydrates back into the diet without even realizing it. Maybe because you've stopped counting carbs, and you're flying it. Or, you may have gone a little too far and convinced yourself that you could invest elsewhere.

While most low-carb plans, such as the Atkins diet and South Beach Diet, encourage you to increase your carbohydrate intake after the induction phase, that doesn't mean you can be less diligent. You still need to follow the guidelines and, if possible, be even more aware of the carbs you're consuming.

To make sure you are within the recommended daily carbohydrate intake:

- Keep a record of everything you eat in a daily diary (and leave nothing).

- Use a carb counter, mobile app, or website to calculate your intake.

- Measure your food as reasonably as possible.

- Look at your portions. It's easy to get carried away by foods that have "just little carbs."

If necessary, you might consider going back to the induction phase and starting all over again—there is no shame in restarting a diet program if it allows you to learn from your mistakes.

Eat According to Your Hunger

While the first or second week of a low-carb diet can be difficult, food cravings that eventually manifest themselves will subside as the body adapts to lower carbohydrate intake.

At this point, if you are eating the right amount of carbohydrates, you will no longer have extreme cravings, but you will go through the normal patterns of hunger and satiety. That's when you're going to have to eat according to your hunger and not by heart.

Eating when you're not hungry only adds carbs you may not need. On the other hand, ignoring your hunger will almost invariably lead you to overeat. As such, it is much better to let hunger signals address your consumption rather than routine.

That said, don't eat three hours before bedtime when your body is less able to burn energy. The same goes for alcohol. At night, your basal metabolism (the rate at which it burns calories at rest) can often slow down to the point where even a small snack can trigger weight gain.

Exercise

Whether you like it or not, you can't sustain weight loss without exercising. While you can certainly lose the first kilos on your diet alone, you're unlikely to maintain the loss if you stay sedentary.

This is why most people who feed on a yo-yo or end up gaining all the weight. When losing weight, basal metabolism will decrease due to reduced food intake. When this happens, you will burn calories more slowly. If you sit around, you almost invariably hit a box when your adapted metabolism barely meets the demands of the foods you're consuming.

One way to combat this is with regular exercise, ideally with strength training. Building lean muscles creates deposits for the energy that the body can fill during rest. Even if you are experiencing fatigue, exercise will trigger the release of hormones, such as endorphins, to improve mood, mental acuity, and energy levels.

Try Ketosis

A ketogenic diet is designed to achieve ketosis, the state in which your body burns more fat and less sugar for energy. The diet is based on a higher intake of healthy fats and a reduction in carbohydrates.

To achieve this state, you may need to reduce carbohydrates drastically. The amount may vary from person to person.

For some, ketosis can be achieved by eating 100 carbohydrates per day. Others require Atkins induction levels.

To find out what's right for you, talk to a qualified nutritionist. Home blood meters are available to measure ketones (by-products of fat metabolism), while reactive urine strips at home can give you a general idea of where you are.

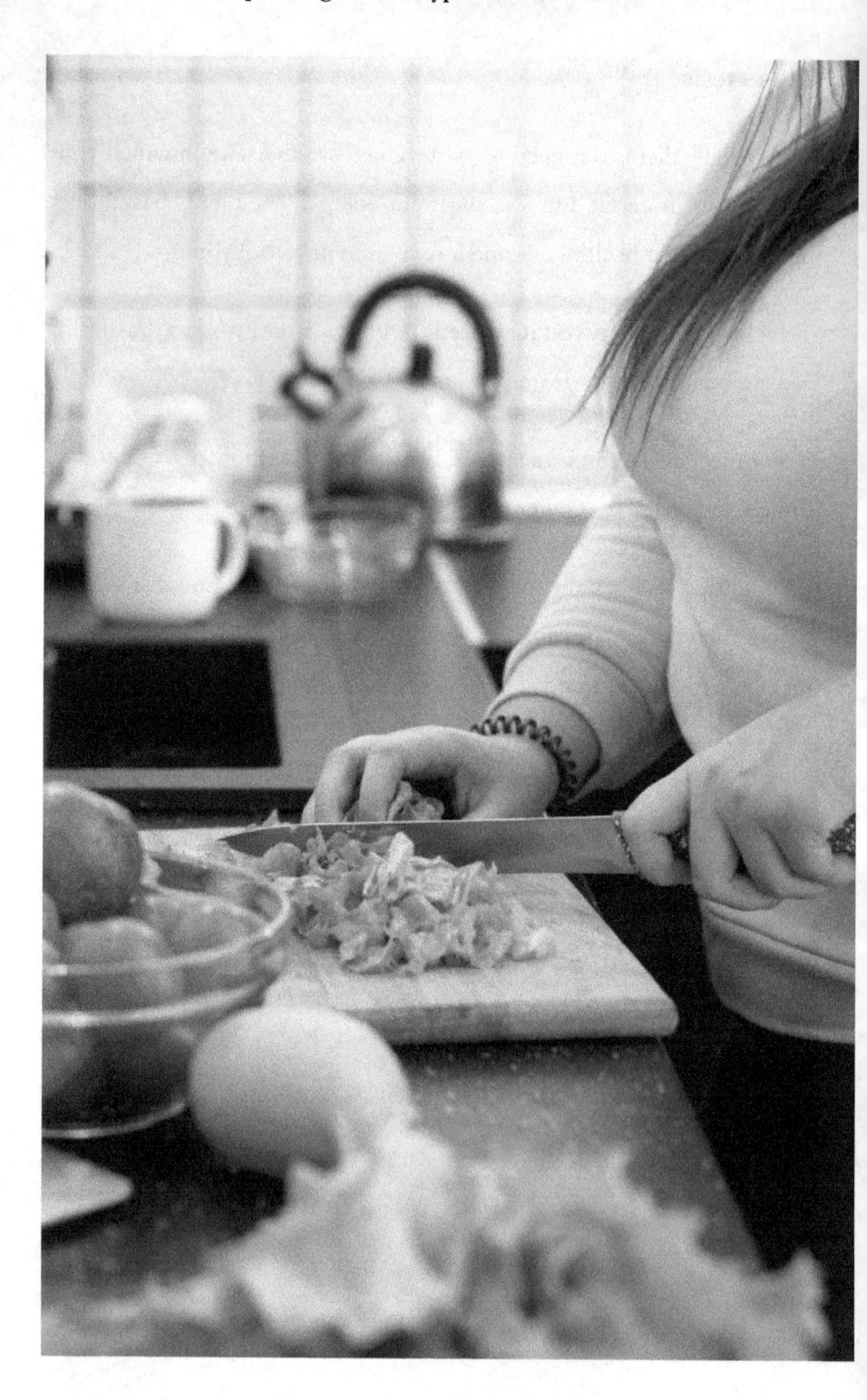

Chapter 5.
First of All, What Is Hypnosis?

Let's start by seeing what hypnosis is NOT. This is not about someone who controls your mind and makes you do ridiculous things while unconscious. Mind control and loss of consciousness—meaning doing something against your will—are the biggest misconceptions about hypnosis.

In reality, hypnosis is precisely the opposite! It is a means that allows you to use your unconscious mind to create the life you have always wanted.

Because of how the entertainment industry portrays hypnotists, people are relieved to see that I'm not wearing a black robe or swinging a watch from a J chain.

Also, you're not unconscious when using hypnosis—it's more like a deep state of relaxation. It is merely the natural, floating sensation you get before falling asleep, or that dreamy feeling you get when you wake up in the morning before being fully aware of where you are and what is around you.

Above all, with hypnosis, it is impossible to push a person to do things against their will, ethics, or sense of decency.

Hypnosis for Weight Loss: Applications and Benefits

Hypnosis for weight loss. When it comes to losing weight, you risk ending up in the usual "free for all" theater: doctors, nutritionists, dieticians, weight-loss gurus, drugs, new age diets, etc.

But there is one thing you may not have thought of yet: asking your unconscious mind for help. Yes, you read that right. Hypnosis for weight loss is based on just that: you're unconscious.

This may surprise you, but no one knows you as well as your unconscious. He knows everything about you. He knows your weaknesses, strengths, and inner conflicts that lead you to have constant nervous hunger, fears, and talents. In short, everything!

Above all, your unconscious is looking forward to activating its powerful resources to make you feel better about yourself. And, at this point, the fateful question arises: how can I ask my unconscious for help?

It's straightforward: you have to ask him in his language, which is a little different than the language we are used to using every day to communicate with friends, colleagues, family, etc.

The unconscious mind speaks a language that can be defined as "analog." It is an idiom made up of symbols, images, sentences structured in a certain way, frequencies, colors, etc. Hypnosis for weight loss is the ideal tool to communicate your intent to lose weight to the unconscious, using its preferred language.

The Benefits of Hypnosis for Weight Loss

Thinking about hypnosis for weight loss might sound a bit bizarre. However, its undoubted advantages must be considered. Here are a few:

- It has no contraindications.

- It is relaxing and anti-stress.

- Increase your willpower.

- It does not introduce chemicals into the body.

- It allows you to achieve goals using YOUR head and not someone else's.

- Once you have learned it, you can use it on your own (self-hypnosis).

So let's see that using hypnosis to lose weight can be a road that can lead you to exciting goals, not only for weight control but also for inner well-being in general.

Hypnosis Increases the Ability to Change

Being in hypnosis makes you more adept at change, which is why hypnosis for weight loss can be useful. It is different from other methods because hypnosis addresses the cause and other unconscious factors that lead a person to overeat. On a subconscious level, there are memories, patterns of habits, fears, emotional associations regarding food, negative beliefs, and the roots of low self-esteem in the minds of each of autism.

But in the unconscious, we also find powerful complementary resources for change and well-being. Hidden treasures ready to make our life healthier and happier.

No other weight loss method addresses the fundamental problems at their root in the way hypnosis does.

But Does Hypnosis Work For Weight Loss?

At this point, we need to be extremely clear. Hypnosis is not the magic bullet that makes you lose weight by continuing to eat recklessly. As we mentioned earlier, hypnosis is a powerful tool to get you back to healthy eating habits and make you follow the dietician's schedule with more incredible willpower (which translates into faster and longer-lasting results).

Early studies from the 1990s found that people who used hypnosis to lose weight lost more than twice the weight than those who dieted without hypnosis or self-hypnosis.

With the seemingly rising cost of prescription drugs, long lists of possible side effects, and the push towards more natural alternatives, hypnosis for weight loss is receiving more and more attention and research as a winning approach to weight loss.

Who Should Use Hypnosis for Weight Loss?

The ideal candidate is, honestly, anyone who has trouble following a healthy diet and exercise program because they can't get over their negative habits. Getting stuck in harmful habits, like eating the whole bag of potato chips instead of stopping when you're full, is a sign of an unconscious problem.

Your subconscious is where your emotions, habits, and addictions are located. Moreover, because hypnosis and self-hypnosis target the subconscious, they can be more effective than just the conscious. Hypnosis has a 93% success rate, with fewer sessions required than psychotherapy and behavioral therapy. This led researchers to find that hypnosis was the most effective way to change habits, thought patterns, and behavior.

Hypnosis for weight loss can also be combined with other natural holistic treatments such as instant emotional release. Hypnosis can also be used as a complement to other weight loss programs designed by professionals to treat various health conditions, be it diabetes, obesity, arthritis, or cardiovascular disease.

How Can I Apply Hypnosis for Weight Loss?

The advice I give to everyone for an optimal path is to start using the self-hypnosis audio against nervous hunger to buy HERE. When you start to get the first results, it is also possible to carry out some individual sessions with the hypnologist live or via video link.

Sessions can vary in length and methodology, depending on the individual characteristics of the client. But in general, you can expect to relax with your eyes closed and let the hypnologist guide you through specific techniques and tips that can help you achieve your goals.

The idea is to train the mind to move towards healthy and away from what is not healthy. Through the client's history, it is possible to determine the unconscious hitches that sent the client out of their original wellness plan. Just as we learn to abuse our bodies with food, we can learn to honor them.

You will experience deep relaxation while being aware of what is being said. Someone describes hypnosis as a condition between being fully awake and asleep, but still alert. You are in full control and can stop the process at any time because you can only be hypnotized if you wish. Hypnosis is a "team effort" to achieve a person's goal.

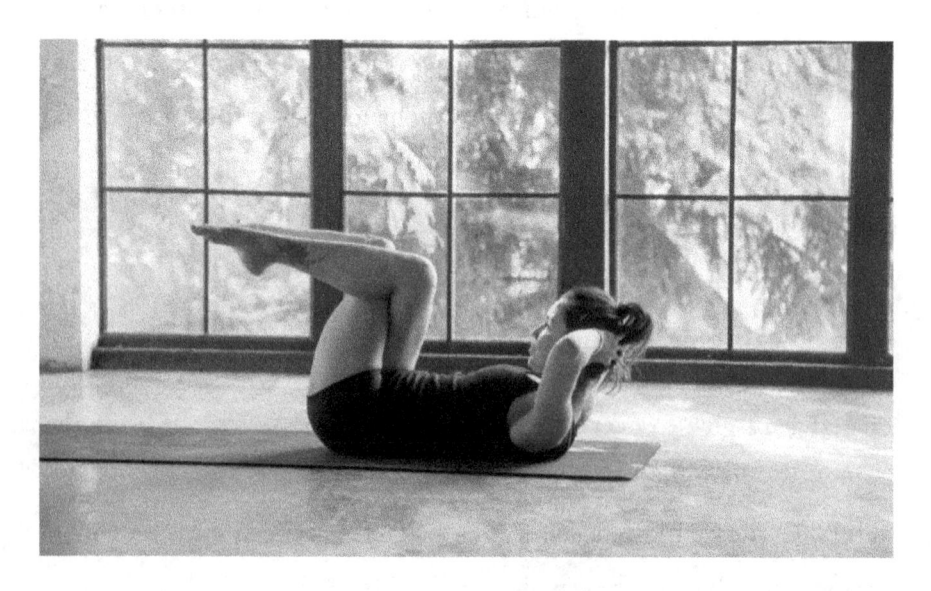

Chapter 6.
Losing Weight with Hypnosis: The Truth about this Practice Spread Abroad

When it comes to losing weight, we turn to nutritionists and dieticians, personal trainers. But, perhaps, you haven't considered hypnosis yet. It turns out that using hypnosis is another avenue that people are venturing in the name of weight loss.

But it's not about someone else controlling your mind and making you do fun things while you're unconscious.

"Mind control and loss of control—or doing something against your will—are the biggest misconceptions about hypnosis," says Kimberly Friedmutter, a hypnotherapist. "Because of how the entertainment industry plays hypnotists, people are relieved to see that I am not wearing a black robe and that I swing a watch from a chain."

Hypnosis as Relaxation

Plus, you're not unconscious when hypnosis occurs—it's more like a deep state of relaxation, explains Fried mutter.

"It is simply the natural, floating feeling you get before falling asleep or that dreamy feeling you get when you wake up in the morning before you are fully aware of where you are and what is around you."

Being in that state makes you more susceptible to change, so hypnosis for weight loss can be useful.

Capri Cruz, psychotherapist, hypnotherapist, and author of Maximize Your Super Powers, says "No other weight loss method addresses fundamental problems at their root the way hypnosis does."

How to Lose Weight through Hypnosis—We Aim For the Goal

How to lose weight with hypnosis? The causes that can lead people to fail to maintain a diet are many. Hypnosis is beneficial in the diet's psychophysical control because it helps prevent binges and support motivation. Let's see in this short guide what are the preliminary indications to follow before starting hypnosis to lose weight

Set the Goal

We need to understand when we ask ourselves how to lose weight with hypnosis is our goal. This is because hypnosis works explicitly on motivation and impulsivity that can cause binges. We will talk about this second point later.

Let's Focus on the Goal

Scientific studies have identified how successful people think when they want to achieve something and have identified some fundamental characteristics of setting a good goal.

So, let's see how a good goal is formulated:

- Let's make it measurable
- Let's limit it in time
- Let's focus on the benefits

Let's Define the Points

To make the goal measurable, we understand, better if with the nutritionist, how much we want to drop. We establish how quickly we will get the desired weight, always better with a nutritionist.

At this point, without being too obsessed with the scale, we will check the weight about every 15 days. For each pound you lose, give yourself a little gratification: you did things right!

- Why do you want to drop? What are the benefits?
- You can do a little imaginative exercise: close your eyes and imagine yourself in the future.

- How will you be with those fewer pounds?

- See yourself with those fewer pounds, what it will be like? And how will others see you?

- How will you perceive your body?

You can repeat this little Exercise every time your motivation drops a little.

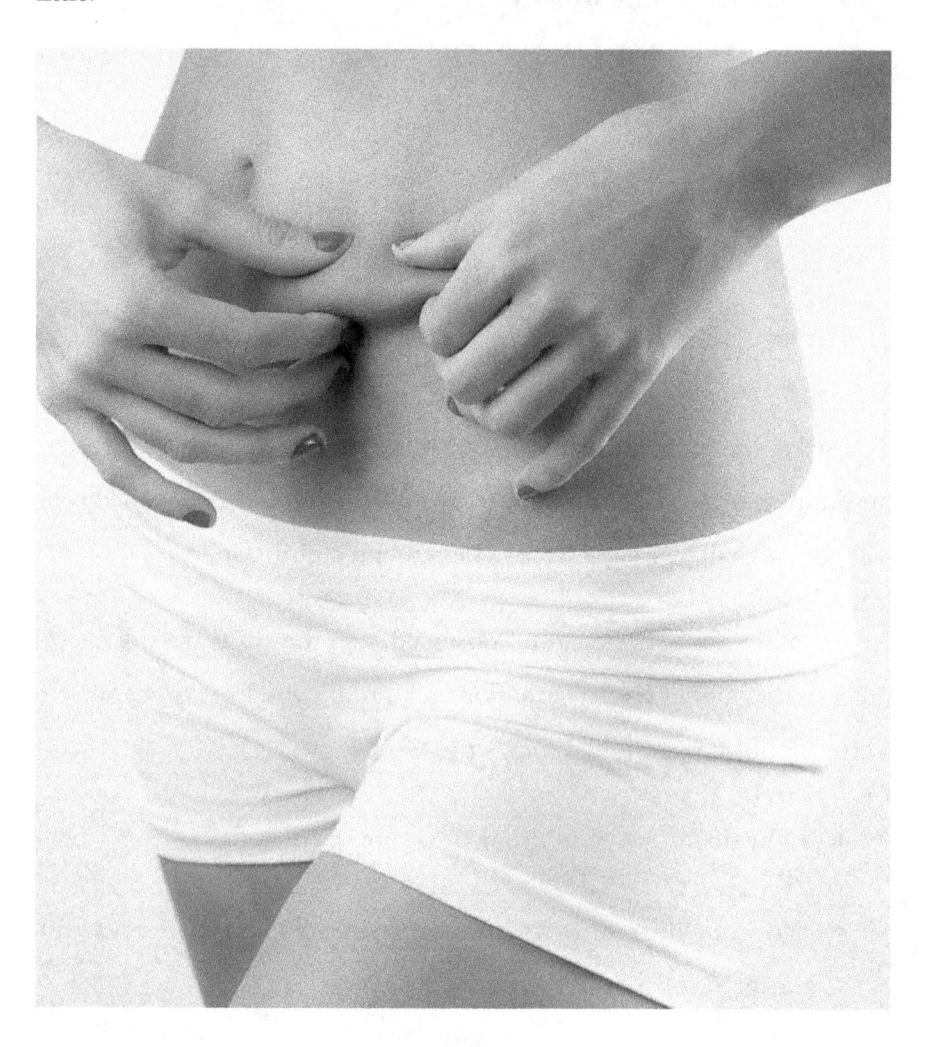

Chapter 7.
Physical Hunger and Emotional Hunger

Throughout our lives, we go through complicated stages in which our stress and anxiety levels exceed the levels to which we are used.

Without realizing it, we look for options to regulate unpleasant sensations such as "food."

Having taken refuge in food at some point in time is not a problem. The problem begins when this becomes a habit.

Whenever I have an emotional need, I turn to food to regulate myself or stabilize myself.

This pattern will generate weight gain and psychological consequences for the person who develops it.

Food in these situations temporarily helps (but DOES NOT SOLVE) to compensate for certain unpleasant emotions and feelings caused by a situation and problem, since when we taste the food, our brain releases many substances (neurotransmitters, including dopamine), which They are responsible for us to feel pleasure.

Once our brain has verified the effectiveness of such food (short-term pleasure), it will look for any opportunity to motivate you to consume that food that produces such good sensations again.

The fact of repeating this behavior (e.g., chocolate intake) over and over again when we feel a negative emotion or sensation will eventually make it a habit.

So, whenever we feel emotionally unstable, we will seek the intake of said food to relieve ourselves.

To begin to solve this problem, we must know how to differentiate the moments in which I am physiologically hungry from those when I am emotionally hungry, and that is why we detail some characteristics that will serve this purpose:

Emotional hunger is sudden, urgent. Also, it is usually selective, thinks about specific foods. It does not generate satiety and usually leads to sadness or guilt.

Physical hunger is gradual, you can wait, and you are open to various food options.

When we feel this hunger, we do achieve the feeling of satiety. That is, eating we pass. Lastly, it does not generate any negative feelings.

In cases where we find it difficult to follow healthy habits, it is advisable to seek help or opinion.

3 Ways to Differentiate Physical Hunger from Emotional

If you have the feeling that you feel hungry all the time, you may be confusing physical hunger with emotional hunger and this is normal because both pangs of hunger can be easily confused.

My experience after several years helping people to incorporate healthier eating habits, both in workshops and individual Mindful Eating sessions, is that one of the great difficulties lies in the fact that it is challenging to differentiate if what they feel is hunger or are other emotions and states manifesting in the body.

Although we can be clear that feeling physical hunger is different from feeling anxiety or stress, the truth is that on many occasions, we give them the same answer, which is to eat.

Eating because of psychological hunger or emotional hunger is a way of eating accompanied by a powerful urge that does not serve to nourish the body. Instead, it has the purpose of comforting, calming, rewarding, distracting, and regulating negative emotions.

According to numerous studies, most people with weight problems have emotional eating patterns without being aware of it.

When we stick to a diet that tells us what and how much to eat, we stop having internal signals of hunger, fullness, and satisfaction, and we begin to function based on the external signals of that diet plan.

After years of dieting, in the end, we are no longer able to know if what we feel is physical hunger or is stress and emotions manifesting in the body.

If you recognize yourself as one of those many people who come home and can't stop snacking until dinner is ready, here are some tips to help you differentiate them, as well as some little tricks to manage them better.

Where It Manifests

Physical hunger manifests itself in the stomach as noise or emptiness and in the body as a feeling of low energy and difficulty concentrating.

On the other hand, when what we feel is emotional hunger, the stomach is calm. However, we can feel some sensations that can be confused with physical hunger, such as a knot in the stomach pit, a feeling of oppression, or restlessness in part lower thorax.

The Type of Food

The second way to differentiate what type of hunger you are focused on the types of food. When we are physically hungry, we are open to several options (fruit, vegetables, meat, eggs, bread, etc.), and if we get famished, any food can be useful for us. Try to remind yourself of feeling ravenous hunger; wouldn't you have eaten anything at the time?

On the other hand, when we feel emotional hunger, we usually have cravings for a particular food, probably with a lump of high sugar, fat, or salt, such as cookies, chocolate, chips, etc. These foods have a pleasant-reinforcing effect on our brains. Therefore, they are the ones that help us calm down or comfort us at that moment.

Therefore, when you feel the urge to eat, stop for a moment and observe what kind of food he is asking you: do you have only one in your head, or can you assess and choose options?

Time

The third way to determine if you are psychologically or physically hungry focuses on time passed since the last meal. If you find yourself looking for food and you had only eaten an hour ago, it's probably emotional hunger.

How to Differentiate and Manage Your Emotional Hunger

1- Close your eyes and try to remember a time when you were starving.

- Where did you feel hunger?
- What physical sensations did you notice in your stomach?

- And in the rest of the body?

- Next, bring your attention to your stomach and your body right now.

- Are you feeling any of those sensations?

2- Also, take your attention to the upper part of your abdomen and thorax and ask yourself:

- Do I feel there any physical sensations that I may be mistaken for hunger?

3- If you find that your stomach is calm, take ten deep and slow breaths, and then ask yourself if you still want to eat.

- This exercise can be more complicated at certain times when physical hunger and emotional hunger are combined, for example, when several hours have passed since the last meal. On top of that, you are accumulating stress. So, both pangs of hunger can make a hard-to-control Molotov cocktail.

4- Do a review of your day to detect those moments in which both types of hunger may be coinciding. Maybe when you get home in the afternoon after a hard day at work or just before your midday meal.

If you detect a repeating pattern, an excellent way to manage them is not to allow both pangs of hunger to reach this critical point:

Make sure that your physical hunger does not reach a level of discomfort, for example, eating some nuts for a while before leaving work. Practice something that relaxes you for a few minutes, such as a little meditation, a hand massage with essential oils, or taking an infusion that you like in small sips. If you want to know more about emotional hunger, I invite you to read this other post where I explain how diets may be creating emotional hunger: Emotional Eating and diet, the cycle from which it is possible to get out.

What Happens to Your Body When You Are Hungry?

Hunger is such a strong instinct that humans go to extremes to satiate it. Hunger is our bodies' way of telling us that it's time to find food, eat, and get on with life. It is a compelling instinct generated when the brain detects changes in hormones and nutrients in the blood. Various signals come from different parts of the digestive system and the bloodstream and some chemical and metabolic factors.

Conclusion

Yoga has proven to be a very positive exercise technique for both body and mind. It increases well-being in many aspects, promoting personal awareness positively, non-competitive group exercise, relaxation, and providing multiple benefits for anyone, especially for eating disorder patients. Therefore, it is recommended that patients with this diagnosis look for this alternative to exercise that they perform regularly or interest both throughout the days.

Moreover, leaving aside for the moment the evidence deriving from the vast world of neuroscience, it is also necessary to clarify whether there are physical and psychic changes that attest to its validity scientifically, beyond the possible individual propensities dictated by "faith" towards a theory or practice.

Weight-loss hypnosis can help you lose a few extra pounds when it's part of a weight loss plan that includes diet, exercise, and counseling. However, it's hard to put it definitively because there's not enough concrete scientific evidence about hypnosis to lose weight only.

Hypnosis is a state of absorption and internal concentration, such as being in a trance. Hypnosis is usually performed with the help of a hypnotherapist through oral repetition and mental imaging.

In general, the best way to lose weight is with diet and exercise. If you've tried dieting and exercise but still have difficulty reaching your weight loss goal, talk to your health care provider about other lifestyle choices or lifestyle changes you can make.

Relying only on weight loss hypnosis probably won't lead to significant weight loss, but using it as a complement to a general lifestyle approach may help explore some people.

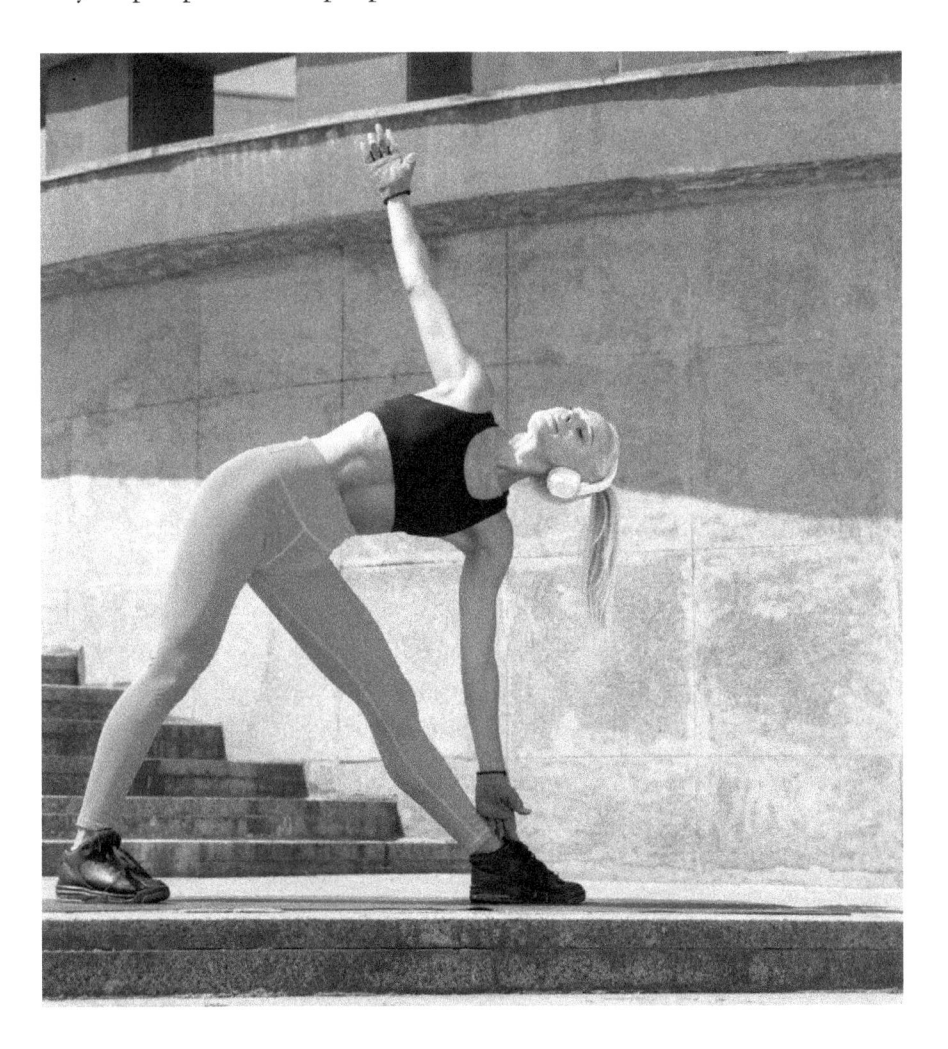

CPSIA information can be obtained
at www.ICGtesting.com
Printed in the USA
BVHW092209080621
609008BV00004B/952

9 781802 998689